Top Nutritional Supplement Buying Guide

Series 1: Health and Wellness

Written by
Daniel Lee Staneart

Contents

Part 1
Places that sell supplements   **6**

      Nutrition Express   7

      ProSource   7

      Swanson Vitamins   8

Part 2
Top supplements and brands to choose   10

      Here's my top twenty safe picks   10 - 53

Part 3
Final Supplement Recommendations   54

      Multivitamin formulas and more   55

Intro to the Supplement Guide

Let's get straight to the point about nutritional supplements. Which supplements, ingredients and brands are the best choices that offer quality and the right price?

Do nutritional supplements really work or provide true results? The answer to that question is yes, based not only on my own personal experience and studies since 1993, but also from thousands of clinical trial studies.

The nutritional supplement industry as a whole is a 35 billion dollar giant and growing. So, since there are so many brands and choices out there for every need what do I choose?

When most people think of supplements they usually think of vitamins, minerals and maybe a few herbs. However, there are so many more beneficial nutritional supplements out there for you to discover for your physical health and well-being.

Part 1

Places that sell supplements

You have many choices where to buy supplements. There are many stores that sell nutritional supplements. Some of the most known retail places to shop are GNC, Vitamin World, The Vitamin Shoppe, Super Supplements, CVS, Walgreens, Rite Aid, Target and even Wal-mart. Discovering which supplements are the best, purest, safest and not harmful definitely takes some research.

There are many online supplement stores available on the internet. Some of the top and my personal favorites that I shop from happen to be wholesale companies. All wholesale nutritional supplement companies sell virtually all known quality brand name supplements as well as their own line of products at a much lower cost than retail.

I try to save more money by shopping for high quality supplement brand names at a much lower wholesale cost. Many times some of the stores listed above, such as GNC, will have some really good sales and bargains as well.

Here are my top three wholesale supplement companies to choose from:

Nutrition Express

Nutrition Express will send you a free catalog by mail or you can go straight to their website. They have a huge selection of quality brand name products as well as their own represented product lines at wholesale prices. Nutrition Express focuses on overall health, weight-loss and muscle building. They also always offer tips, advice and have excellent articles. Here is their toll free number and website link: 1-800-338-7979 or go to

www.nutritionexpress.com

ProSource

ProSource supplements will send you a free catalog by mail or you can go straight to their website. They have a good selection of quality brand name products as well as their own high quality product line at wholesale prices. ProSource focuses more on muscle building and weight-loss. They also always offer tips, advice, excellent articles and helpful supplement ratings. Here is their toll free number and website link: 1-800-310-1555 or go to www.prosource.net

Swanson Vitamins

Swanson Vitamins will send you a free catalog by mail or you can go straight to their website. They primarily focus on their own Swanson name products, but also have a great selection of quality brand name products at wholesale prices. Swanson Vitamins is a great company for finding unique and herbal supplements and they tend to focus on overall health. They also have good supplement articles, informative videos and customer reviews. Here is their toll free number and website link: 1-800-437-4148 or go to www.swansonvitamins.com

This supplement buying guide is part of a 3-book series. This is series 1, which will focus on health and wellness supplements that offer and provide overall good health and benefits.

Series 2 will be about muscle building, which will list top supplements for that category, and of course Series 3 will focus on weight loss. All three books are top nutritional supplement buying guides.

Hopefully this guide will give you direction in finding the right supplement, brand and price for your needs. I wrote this book to help people and to answer these three questions .... What, Where and How much?

Remember to always consult your doctor before using certain supplements especially if you're taking medications.

Let's get started....

Part 2

Top supplements and brands to choose

What are some of the top nutritional supplements and brands to choose this new 2016 year to benefit your health, especially based on effectiveness, quality and price?

Here's my top twenty safe picks

1. Turmeric (Curcuma longa): Turmeric is a yellow colored Indian spice commonly used in curry and even mustard. You can find the cooking spice itself in various retail and grocery stores such as Wal-mart. The active chemical ingredient in turmeric is curcumin, also known as curcuminoids. They are very powerful phytochemicals, natural polyphenols, antioxidants and anti-inflammatory agents. This spice works excellent in fighting free radicals and inflammation in the body such as arthritis.

Turmeric offers such a wide array of health benefits for joints, skin, stomach, blood, liver and heart health. Other great benefits include anti-cancer, anti-allergen, anti-viral and anti-bacterial properties, healthy weight loss, increased sex drive and possibly fertility plus more. This spice has also been shown to be beneficial for weight loss after pregnancy.

What are some of the best Turmeric (Curcumin) supplement brands to use?

When purchasing supplements I look for quality and price. Keep in mind that I recommend purchasing from wholesale companies such as Nutrition Express. I will say though that it is very convenient to go down to your local nutrition store such as GNC and pick products up, especially if you need it that day.

Here are my top brands to choose from for buying Turmeric (Curcumin): NOW Foods, Jarrow Formulas, Nature's Way, Solaray, Doctor's Best and Lindberg. The wholesale price ranges from 9 to 32 dollars for about 60 to 180 caps/tabs.

There is a turmeric supplement brand called Radiance that I picked up at a convenient local CVS for only about 12 dollars. It definitely works and I could tell a difference, so it is good quality at a decent price.

A good tip for increasing the absorption and bio-availability of turmeric (curcumin) is to combine or take it with meals or supplements containing oils (healthy fats), cayenne, black pepper and even bromelain, an enzyme found in pineapples.

One supplement that I take with turmeric is ginger which seems to offer more health benefits and possibly better absorption. Turmeric itself is a member of the ginger family.

Turmeric and curcumin are my top "go to" supplements. Some other strong potent curcumin formulas containing the C3 complex or phytosome technology featuring meriva are backed by some impressive clinical trials. Some high quality brands offer both of these potent types of curcumin formulas. NOW Foods brand offers a supplement containing both turmeric and bromelain for better absorption.

My top picks for supplemental turmeric and curcumin based on quality and price:

NOW Foods brand Curcumin with 60 vcaps 665 mg standardized to 95% curcuminoids for $14.99. Purchase online through Nutrition Express

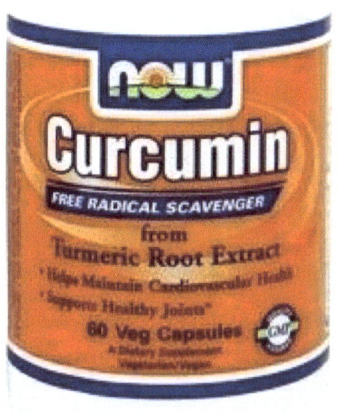

Jarrow Formulas Curcumin 95 with 60 caps 500 mg containing 95% curcuminoids for $13.95 through Nutrition Express

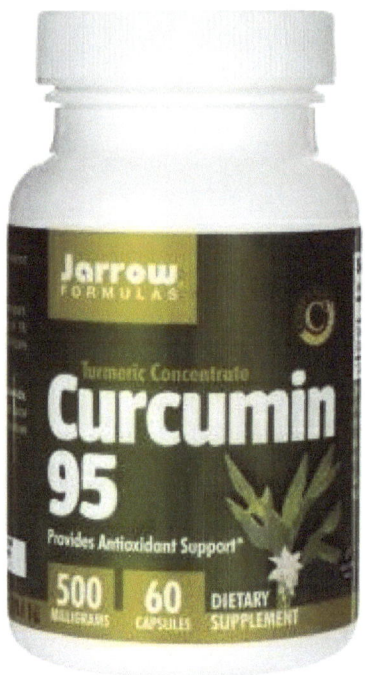

I will say once again that I'm very pleased with the Radiance brand turmeric product I purchased at my local CVS for $11.99 with 100 caps at 400 mg. However, this turmeric is not a standardized (extract) product.

2. Ginger (Zingiber officinale): Ginger is a flowering plant whose underground stem (rhizome) is used as a spice and natural medicine. Ginger root is widely used for motion sickness, stomach problems, joint pain and even may reduce cancer risk.

Here are some good ginger root supplemental brands to choose from: Nature's Way, NOW Foods, Jarrow Formulas, Oregon's Wild Harvest, Lindberg and even Swanson from Swanson Vitamins or Radiance from your local CVS. Wholesale prices range between 4 to 6 dollars while retail runs about 7 to 9 dollars all providing 30 to 180 caps.

My top picks for supplemental Ginger Root based on quality and price:

Nature's Way brand Ginger Root with 100 caps 550 mg for $4.40. Purchase online through Swanson Vitamins or same product from Nutrition Express for $5.49

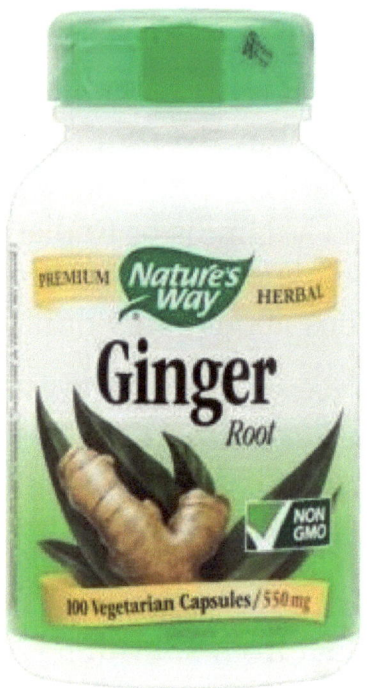

You can purchase Nature's Way brand at GNC for $8.99, which is where I normally pick up this product instead of waiting on mail order.

3. Hawthorn (Crataegus): Hawthorn is an herbal plant whose leaves, berries and flowers are used to make medicine. Hawthorn (Hawthorn extract) is used for heart and blood vessel health. It is sometimes used for stomach or skin problems as well. Hawthorn actually does help lower blood pressure.

Remember to always consult your doctor before using certain supplements especially if you're taking medications. For the most part, good quality supplements are safe to take under any circumstance especially when using the right recommended product and right amount. Do your own research and get advice if you're not sure.

Here are some good brands to choose from for Hawthorn: Solaray, Lindberg, NOW Foods, Nature's Way and Swanson. Price ranges from 4 to 10 dollars providing 60 to 180 caps.

NOW Foods offers a blood pressure health supplement containing Hawthorn and Grape Seed extract that would be very beneficial costing about 15 dollars for 90 caps.

My top pick for supplemental Hawthorn (Hawthorn extract) based on quality and price:

Solaray brand Hawthorn extract with 60 caps 100 mg extract with 225 mg berry for $3.59. Purchase online through Nutrition Express

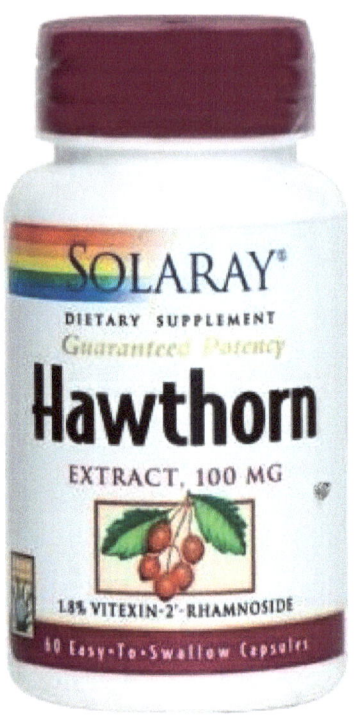

4. Grape Seed Extract (Vitis Vinifera): Grape seed extract is a derivative of grape seeds or more simply put...it comes from grapes. The supplemental form of this contains very powerful free-radical fighting antioxidant compounds such as polyphenols, anthocyanins and oligomeric proanthocyanidins among other chemicals.

It is widely used for heart and cardiovascular health. Grape seed is also beneficial for blood pressure, immune system, skin, eyes, joints and has potential cancer fighting properties.

Here are some good brands to choose from: Nature's Way, NOW Foods, Lindberg, Swanson and Olympian Labs. Prices range from 6 to 25 dollars providing 30 to 240 caps. Many high quality brands like Solaray, Jarrow Formulas and Nature's Way produce supplements providing healthy benefits with a combination of ingredients that will include grape seed extract.

My top picks for supplemental Grape Seed Extract based on quality and price:

NOW Foods brand Grape Seed with 90 vcaps 60 mg extract along with 300 mg citrus bioflavonoids for $7.62. Purchase online through Swanson Vitamins

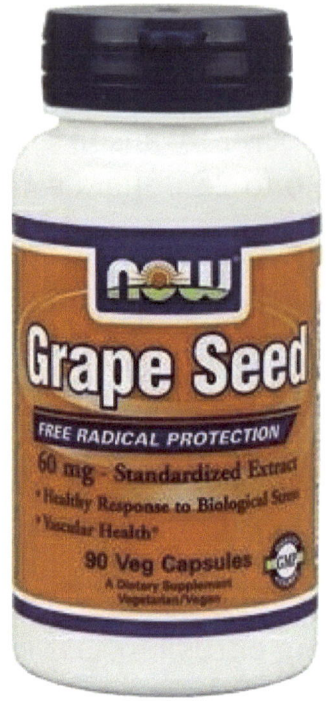

Lindberg brand also offers a high quality fair priced product as well for only $6.49 through Nutrition Express

5. Krill Oil: Krill Oil is extracted from small krill fish crustaceans (shellfish) found in the ocean. Krill Oil contains an excellent source of omega-3 fatty acids and astaxanthin, which is a very powerful antioxidant. This type of supplement is very beneficial for the heart, joints, skin and immune system. Astaxanthin has very strong free radical fighting properties.

Here are some good brands to choose from: NOW Foods, Lindberg, Nature's Way and Swanson. Price ranges from 10 to 70 dollars providing 30 to 180 softgels.

My top pick for supplemental Krill Oil based on quality and price:

NOW Foods brand Neptune Krill Oil with 60 softgels 500 mg also containing phospholipids and astaxanthin for $18.19. Purchase online through Nutrition Express

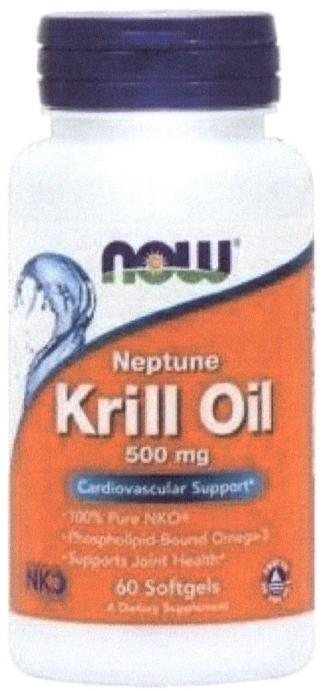

6. Cilantro (Coriandrum Sativum): Cilantro are leaves from the coriander plant. Cilantro leaves, which are full of nutrients, are a popular culinary herb used in Mexican dishes. They are powerful free radical fighters and provide health benefits for the stomach and intestinal tract.

It's not very easy to find a cilantro supplement, but Swanson Vitamins does produce a good quality one from its own Swanson line of products.

I personally like to eat cilantro. My wife often prepares and cooks Mexican food and so she always buys fresh cilantro and uses it very generously.

My top pick for supplemental Cilantro based on quality and price:

Swanson Vitamins brand Cilantro with 60 caps 425 mg for $3.89. Purchase online through Swanson Vitamins

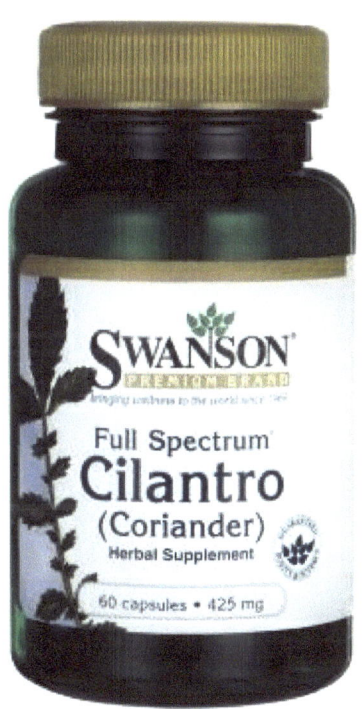

7. NAC (N-Acetyl Cysteine): NAC is a sulfur containing amino acid. It's a precursor to the body's production of glutathione, which is our body's primary cellular antioxidant. N-Acetyl Cysteine is a powerful antioxidant used for its fatigue and disease fighting properties as well as liver, lung and cardiovascular health.

Here are some good brands to choose from: NOW Foods, Swanson, Lindberg, Jarrow Formulas and Doctor's Best.

My top pick for supplemental NAC based on quality and price:

NOW Foods brand NAC with 100 vcaps 600 mg containing small amounts of molybdenum and selenium for $13.04. Purchase online through Swanson Vitamins

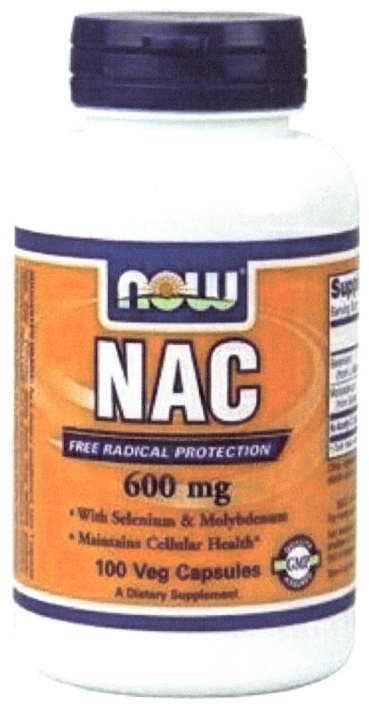

Lindberg brand NAC with 120 vcaps 600 mg also containing small amounts of the trace minerals selenium and molybdenum for $11.99. Purchase online through Nutrition Express

8. Olive Leaf Extract: This powerful extract of course comes from olive leaves but contains a strong free radical fighting antioxidant known as Oleuropein. Olive Leaf Extract is widely used for both cardiovascular and immune system health. It may also be beneficial for blood sugar maintenance. This is a great health supplement to use but olive oil itself still has many confirmed health benefits.

Here are some good brands to choose from: NOW Foods, Swanson, Lindberg, Nature's Way, Natural Factors and Planetary Herbals. It's best to buy a product that contains 12 to 20% standardized oleuropein. However, some high quality brands like NOW Foods contain 6%.

There is one new olive leaf extract product from NOW Foods that contains 18% extract with 50 vcaps 400 mg and 100 mg of Echinacea angustifolia extract for even more immune boosting power for $9.63 through Swanson Vitamins.

My top picks for supplemental Olive Leaf Extract based on quality and price:

Lindberg Olive Leaf with 60 caps 500 mg for $7.99 through Nutrition Express

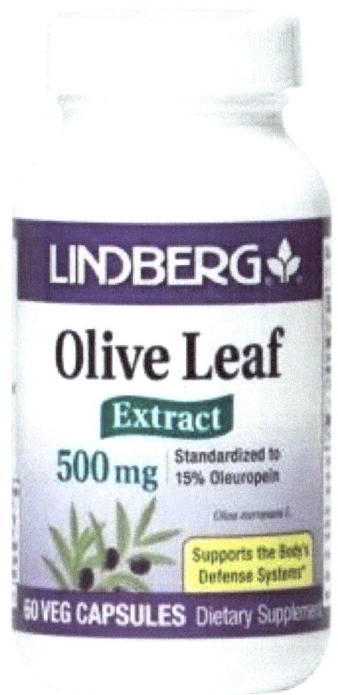

Nature's Way Olive Leaf with 60 caps 250 mg extract and 180 mg olive leaf for $7.09 through Swanson Vitamins

Swanson brand Olive Leaf Extract Super Strength with 60 caps 750 mg through Swanson Vitamins for $9.49

The NOW Foods brand olive leaf extract with 50 vcaps 400 mg and 100 mg echinacea is definitely recommended if you can find it in stock.

9. White Willow Bark (Salix Alba): White willow bark is nature's natural aspirin. It contains a compound called Salicin and is used widely to reduce inflammation, pain and swelling in the body and joints. This supplement is a great alternative to pain medicine but without side effects and promotes true healing.

Here are some good brands to choose from: Solaray, Nature's Way, NOW Foods and Swanson.

My top pick for supplemental White Willow Bark based on quality and price:

Solaray brand White Willow Bark with 100 caps 400 mg for $5.19. Purchase online through Nutrition Express

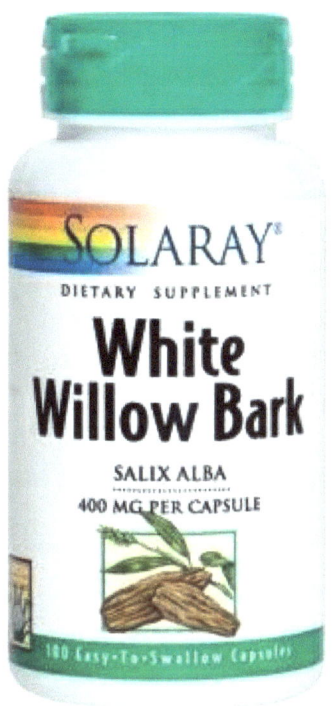

Swanson Vitamins also offers a good customer rated product. It's called Swanson Maximum Strength White Willow Bark containing 25% salicin with 60 vcaps 500 mg for $4.99

10. Pycnogenol (Pinus maritimer or pinaster): Pycnogenol is a powerful extract from pine bark, specifically French Maritime Pine Bark, that contains flavonoids and other potent antioxidants such as procyanidins that fight free radicals. It is used for heart, circulatory, joint, skin, connective tissue, eye and blood sugar health. Pine bark extract also has anti-inflammatory properties and sexual enhancement benefits.

Here are some good brands to choose from: NOW Foods, Nature's Way, Lindberg, Swanson and Country Life.

My top pick for supplemental Pycnogenol based on quality and price:

NOW Foods brand Pycnogenol with 60 caps 30 mg for $17.99. Purchase online through Swanson Vitamins

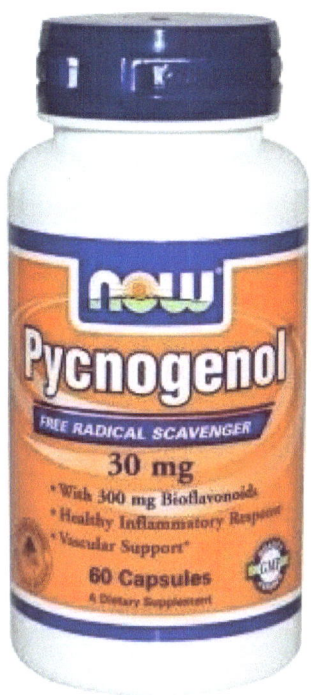

Nature's Way also offers a good quality Pycnogenol product with 30 tabs 50 mg and added Vitamin E for better absorption for only $12.98. You can also purchase it online through Swanson Vitamins.

11. Cinnamon Bark (Cinnamomum Verum or Zeylanicum): True safe cinnamon, known as Ceylon Cinnamon, comes from a small evergreen tree that is native to Southeast Asia, specifically Sri-Lanka. Cinnamon has been used as a spice and healing medicine for centuries. The cinnamon you find on grocery store shelves in powder form and in some food products is primarily Cassia Cinnamon (Cinnamon Aromaticum), also known as Chinese or Saigon cinnamon. This type of cinnamon contains an ingredient called coumarin, which in high amounts can be toxic to the liver and kidneys.

When using cinnamon frequently in your diet or if you're looking for a cinnamon supplement, try to find and buy organic cinnamon bark powder or Ceylon Cinnamon (Cinnamomum Verum). Organic forms of cinnamon bark in supplement form seem to be safe even if they contain some cassia form of cinnamon, but I still recommend the ceylon form.

What are the benefits of cinnamon bark (true cinnamon)?

Provides blood sugar health and known to lower blood sugar in people with type II diabetes. It can lower blood pressure as well as provide skin, metabolism, immune system, teeth, digestive, weight loss, muscle, sexual, circulatory and brain health. It contains some antioxidants and has anti-bacterial, anti-microbial and age defying properties. It also has potential to protect the brain from Alzheimer's disease.

It seems that supplementing cinnamon with a liver protecting herb like Milk Thistle would be a great idea as well.

Here are some good brands to choose from containing true ceylon cinnamon (cinnamon verum): Solaray, Oregon's Wild Harvest and Swanson. Other brands that carry cinnamon bark, even with extract, may contain cassia cinnamon but still can be beneficial .... just don't take too much. These other brands are NOW Foods, Nature's Way, Lindberg and Doctor's Best.

My top picks for supplemental Cinnamon Bark (Cinnamon Verum) from Ceylon based on quality and price:

Solaray Cinnamon Bark with 60 caps 500 mg for $5.19. Purchase online through Nutrition Express

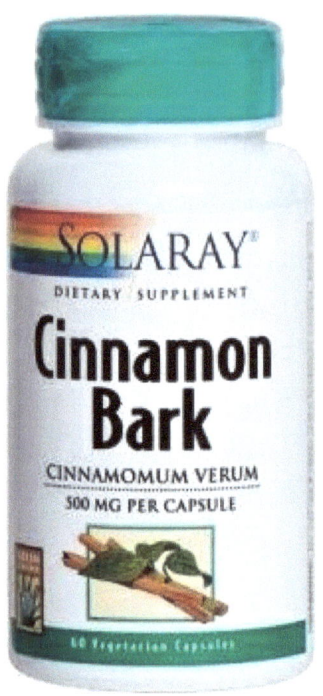

Swanson's brand True Cinnamon Full Spectrum with 90 caps 600 mg for $5.99. Purchase online through Swanson Vitamins

12. Milk Thistle (Silybum marianum): Milk thistle is a flowering plant that has been used for over 2,000 years, especially for liver and gall bladder health. There are many clinical studies involving milk thistle and liver health. The active ingredient in milk thistle is Silymarin which comes from the seeds of milk thistle. This excellent detoxifying herb and extract has also been used to treat some diseases.

Here are some good brands to choose from: NOW Foods, Jarrow Formulas, Solaray, Nature's Way, Lindberg, Swanson and Nature's Plus.

My top picks for supplemental Milk Thistle based on quality and price:

NOW Foods Silymarin Milk Thistle Extract (double strength) with 100 caps 300 mg standardized to 80% with added Dandelion root and Artichoke for $13.99. Purchase online through Nutrition Express

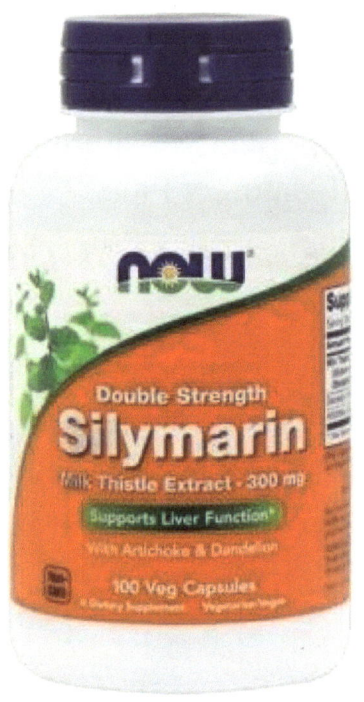

Here are more recommended brands for Milk Thistle:

NOW Foods Silymarin Extract with 120 caps 150 mg standardized to 80% with added Turmeric for $9.69 also through Nutrition Express

Jarrow Formulas Milk Thistle Standardized Silymarin Extract 30:1 and 80% flavonoids with 200 caps 150mg for $12.79. Purchase online through Swanson Vitamins

Swanson's brand Milk Thistle (standardized) with 120 caps 250 mg standardized to 80% Silymarin for $6.69. Purchase online through Swanson Vitamins

You can also conveniently pick up a good quality milk thistle supplement from CVS from their Radiance brand of products for $13.99.

13. Nettle Root "Stinging Nettle" (Urtica Dioica): Nettle (root or leaf) is a herb and small plant that grows in various areas including the United States. It has been used for over 2,000 years for its health benefits. Stinging Nettle is widely used for allergies, hayfever, joint pain as well as respiratory, prostate and sexual health.

It also has testosterone boosting potential as well as anti-inflammatory and free radical fighting properties. Stinging Nettle root and extracts seem to be the most potent and beneficial.

Here are some good brands to choose from: NOW Foods, Nature's Way, Oregon's Wild Harvest, Solaray and Swanson.

My top pick for supplemental Stinging Nettle based on quality and price:

NOW Foods Stinging Nettle Root Extract with 90 vcaps 500 mg (250 mg extract) for $7.99. Purchase online through Nutrition Express

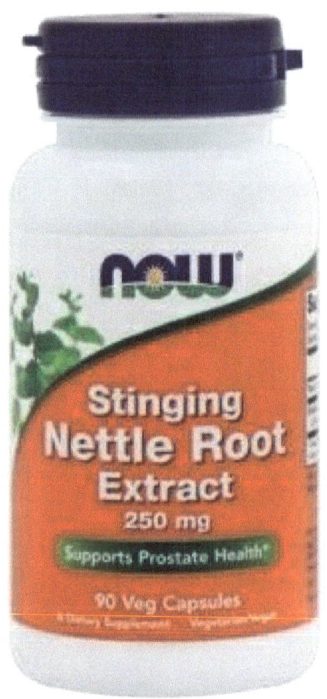

14. Valerian Root (Valeriana Officinalis): Valerian Root is a herb that comes from a flowering plant. This herb is widely used for health relaxation and sleep benefits. It does actually work and helps to provide a more restful night without side effects. Valerian root extracts containing Valerenic Acids seem to be the most potent and work the best.

Here are some good brands to choose from: Nature's Way, Lindberg, NOW Foods and Swanson.

My top pick for supplemental Valerian Root Extract based on quality and price:

Nature's Way Valerian Standardized Extract with 90 caps 400 mg with 110 mg extract at 0.8% valerenic acids for $6.59. Purchase online through Swanson Vitamins

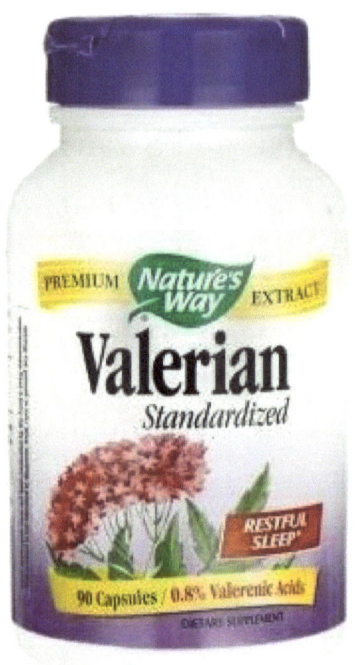

NOW Foods carries a high quality brand of Valerian Root Extract in liquid form containing 1:2 tincture strength with 37 servings or cut the dose in half and you'll have 74 servings all for $9.19. You can purchase online through Swanson Vitamins.

You can also conveniently pick up Nature's Way brand Valerian Extract at both GNC and CVS between 11 and 12 dollars.

It would also be beneficial to purchase a good quality

L-Tryptophan supplement to take with Valerian root to really increase health benefits and restful sleep. L-Tryptophan is an essential amino acid and precursor to melatonin and seratonin which are important hormones for mood and stress regulation. It can also reduce carbohydrate cravings.

A good recommendation for L-Tryptophan supplementation would be to choose a product from these brands: NOW Foods, Lindberg, Jarrow Formulas, Doctor's Best or Swanson.

Lindberg's brand of L-Tryptophan offers (USP) pure grade with 60 caps 500 mg for $10.99 through Nutrition Express.

15. Andrographis (Andrographis Paniculata): Andrographis is an ancient herb that has been used for centuries for healing and immune support fighting off flu and colds among other health benefits. This is a very powerful herb and so dietary supplements have been becoming more available for it. When purchasing this in supplement form look for a full spectrum product with extract.

Here are some good brands to choose from: Nature's Way, NOW Foods, Planetary Herbals and Swanson.

My top pick for supplemental Andrographis based on quality and price:

Nature's Way Andrographis Standardized with 60 vcaps 400 mg from which 300 mg is extract standardized to 10% andrographpholides for $7.39. Purchase online through Swanson Vitamins

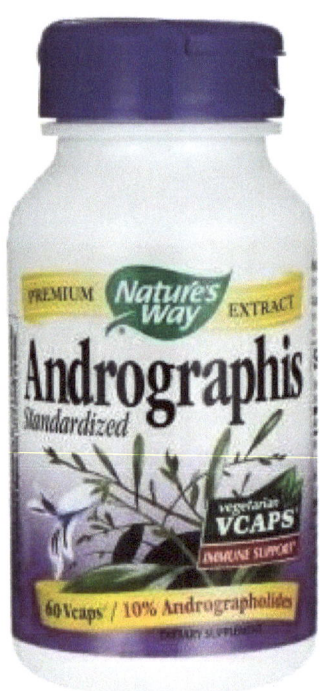

16. Phosphatidylserine (PS): Phosphatidylserine is a special chemical particularly involved with the brain.

It is widely used in supplement form to improve memory, focus, mood, relaxation, cognitive function and stress health. Phosphatidylserine also has potential to combat Alzheimer's disease, ADHD and depression. It may also improve athletic performance.

Here are some good brands to choose from: NOW Foods, Nature's Way, Jarrow Formulas, Lindberg, Source Naturals, Swanson and Doctor's Best. Some of these are made using soybean oil and some are soy-free so it just depends on which you prefer.

My top pick for supplemental Phosphatidylserine based on quality and price:

Jarrow Formulas Phosphatidylserine PS100 with 60 sgels 100 mg for $18.99. This product is soy-free non-GMO and you can purchase it online through Swanson Vitamins

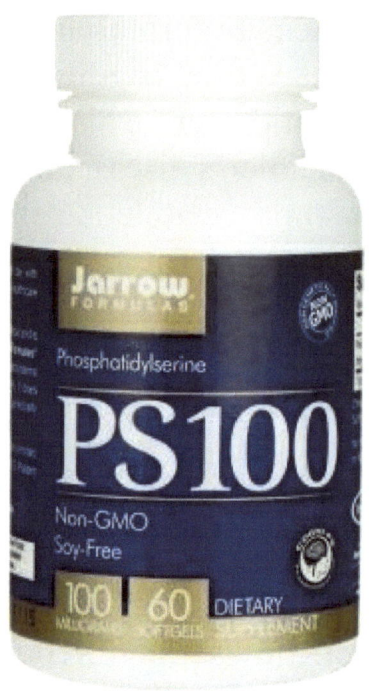

17. Garlic (Allium Sativum): Most people know what garlic is all about, but not everyone knows all about its health benefits. Garlic produces a powerful chemical called Allicin It has medicinal and anti-bacterial properties. It is used widely for immune, heart, circulatory, blood pressure, intestinal, digestive, blood sugar and liver health. Garlic is also known for treating a whole host of ailments including hemorrhoids and various cancers such as colon cancer.

Here are some good brands to choose from: Kyolic (Wakunaga), Nature's Way, Kyoto, NOW Foods, Swanson and Lindberg. All these brands are good quality, but for many years Kyolic has specialized in garlic supplements and they are supreme. They are really known for producing high quality aged and odor-less garlic products even in combination with other beneficial ingredients.

There is speculation as to whether aged garlic is as potent as standard garlic. However, both offer great health benefits backed my many clinical studies, claims and personal testimonies.

My top picks for supplemental Garlic based on quality and price:

Kyolic Reserve Aged Garlic Extract with 120 caps 600 mg for $14.79. No odor or after taste. Purchase online through Swanson Vitamins. You can also buy this product with 60 caps for $9.49

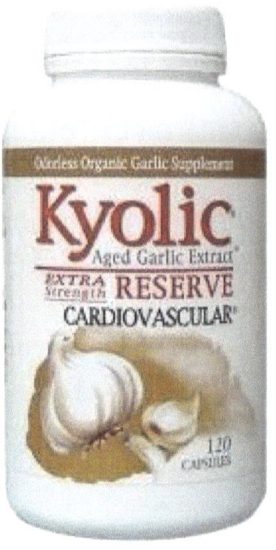

Nature's Way Garlicin Cardio Odor-free Garlic with 90 smart release enteric-coated tabs 350 mg releasing 3,200 mcg for $9.94 through Swanson Vitamins

NOW Foods Odorless Garlic with 100 sgels 50 mg concentrated extract for $6.29 through Swanson Vitamins

Lindberg 500 mg Odorless Garlic with 120 sgels 500 mg and 5 mg of an 100:1 extract for $5.99 through Nutrition Express

Swanson Kyoto Aged Black Garlic (naturally fermented) with 30 caps 650 mg for $11.99 through Swanson Vitamins

18. Alpha Lipoic Acid (ALA): Alpha Lipoic Acid is a fatty acid produced naturally in the body and found in certain foods. It is also a universally powerful fat and water soluble antioxidant protecting both the inside and outside of the cell. It even enhances the power of other antioxidants. The supplement form of ALA is used widely for fighting free radicals as well as providing glutathione synthesis and boosting energy.

ALA also provides and supports liver, weight management, kidney, cardiovascular, glucose metabolism and immune health. There is strong evidence and studies that it can help people with type II diabetes, nerve damage and even cancer. It also has potential to fight against dementia.

Alpha Lipoic Acid may lower blood sugar levels, so be aware especially if you have diabetes or hypoglycemia.

Here are some good brands to choose from: Jarrow Formulas, NOW Foods, Doctor's Best, Healthy Origins, Nature's Way, Lindberg and Swanson.

***My top pics for supplemental Alpha Lipoic Acid
based on quality and price:***

NOW Foods Alpha Lipoic Acid with 60 vcaps 100
mg including vitamins C and E for $7.67. You can
purchase online through Swanson Vitamins

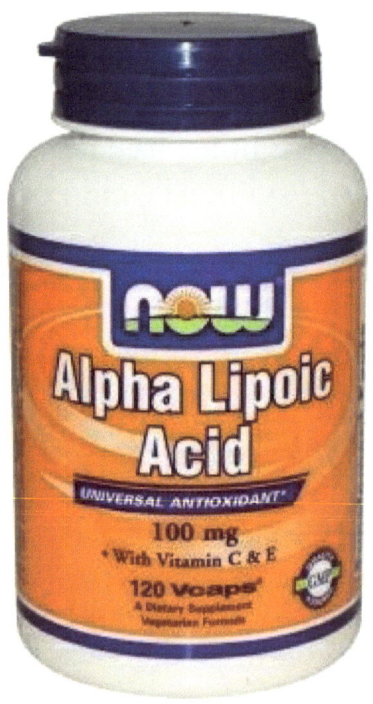

Nature's Way Alpha Lipoic Acid Plus Rosemary with
60 caps 50 mg and 310 mg rosemary for $12.09

through Swanson Vitamins

Jarrow Formulas R-Alpha Lipoic Acid with Biotin providing 100 caps 100 mg and 150 mcg d-biotin for $16.89 through Nutrition Express

19. Boswellia (Boswellia Serrata): Boswellia is a medium sized plant-like tree that produces an extract and resin known as the biblical frankincense. It contains powerful terpenoids called boswellic acids that are extremely beneficial. Boswellia extract is a widely used herb with anti-inflammatory properties backed by clinical studies. It is used as a treatment for asthma, arthritis, joint health, pain and potentially even depression when used as an incense. It is even used for patients undergoing cancer treatments.

Here are some good brands to choose from: Nature's Way, Solaray, NOW Foods, Nature's Answer, Nature's Plus and Swanson.

My top pics for supplemental Boswellia based on quality and price:

Nature's Way Boswellia Standardized Extract with 60 tabs 307 mg containing 65% Boswellic Acids for $6.95. Purchase online through Swanson Vitamins.

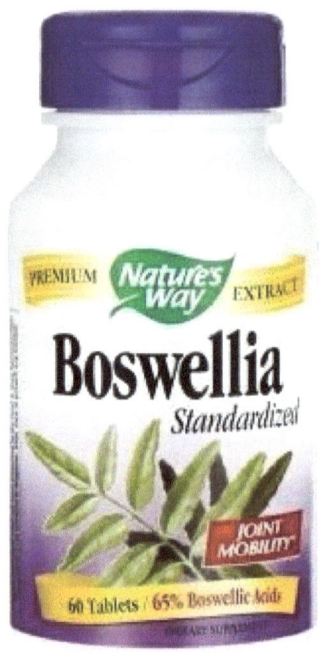

NOW Foods Boswellia Extract with 90 sgels 500 mg containing 65% Boswellic Acids for $15.93 through Swanson Vitamins

NOW Foods Boswellia Extract with 120 vcaps with 250 mg containing 65% Boswellic Acids with added Turmeric Root Extract and powder containing 95% curcuminoids for $16.69 through Swanson Vitamins

Solaray Boswellia with 60 caps 300 mg containing

65% Boswellic Acids with added Devil's Claw 125 mg for $11.89 through Swanson Vitamins

20. Ashwagandha (Withania Somnifera): Ashwagandha is one of the oldest known medicinal herbs. It's a plant, and of course herb, that is an adaptogen containing alkaloids. This special herb has been widely used for centuries providing energy, relaxation and stress relief. It also benefits and provides mood, emotional, brain, muscular, weight management, nervous system, immune and joint health.

Here are some good brands to choose from: Nature's Way, Jarrow Formulas, NOW Foods, Solaray, Himalaya Herbal Healthcare, Life Extension, Planetary Herbals, Lindberg and Swanson.

My top picks for supplemental Ashwagandha based on quality and price:

Jarrow Formulas Ashwagandha with root extract 120 caps 300 mg containing extract called KSM-66 providing min. 8% withanolide glycosides (withanolides) for $13.54. Purchase online through Swanson Vitamins

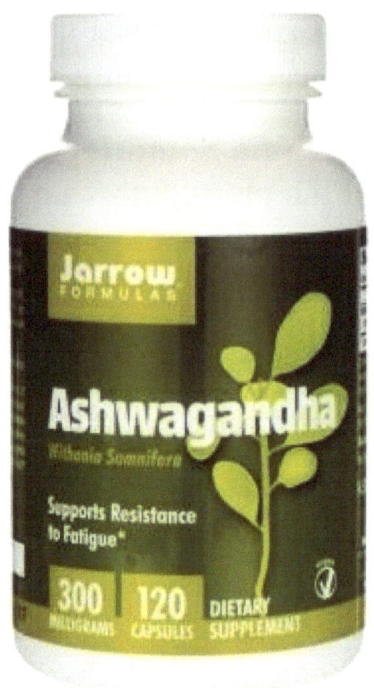

NOW Foods Ashwagandha with 90 vcaps 450 mg containing root extract providing 2.5% withanolides for $8.78 through Swanson Vitamins

Nature's Way Ashwagandha Standardized with 60 caps 500 mg containing root extract providing 2.5% withanolides for $9.73 through Swanson Vitamins

Lindberg Ashwagandha 125 mg Sensoril patented formula with 60 caps 125 mg containing root extract providing 10% withanolide glycoside conjugates for

$5.99 through Nutrition Express
Swanson Ashwagandha Extract with 60 caps 450 mg containing extract providing 1.0% alkaloids and 1.5% withanolides for $4.99 through Swanson Vitamins

In conclusion, this top twenty list of supplements are specifically selected for best overall health and wellness catering to many needs. Keep in mind as well that many diseases and health problems begin in the digestive system, so what you take, ingest and eat will make a significant difference in your overall health.

Part 3

Final supplement recommendations

No matter what doctors or even the media may say, nutritional supplements can offer great health benefits for everyone. Using good quality supplements in the right amounts will definitely bring you healing and healthy results.

Once again, remember to always consult your doctor before using nutritional supplements especially if you're taking medications, specifically meds for the heart, blood pressure and diabetes.

What do I think about Multivitamin/mineral supplements?

I think that many of them are harmful and toxic, because of the use of synthetic ingredients along with bad combinations of ingredients that can even counteract each other. There are reports of humans being harmed and receiving toxicity from synthetic ingredients, which can slowly hinder the bodies health.

Synthetic vitamins and minerals are "mimics" of the true natural form. They are scientifically created in a lab and contain chemical compounds that are not healthy at all for human consumption. Even some standalone vitamin or mineral supplements and prenatal formulas are synthetically made so the brand and quality you choose does make a difference.

The best type of "multivitamin" supplements are the ones that contain full-spectrum naturally occurring ingredients in the right combination from all natural sources. Also, a vitamin/mineral supplement from whole food sources are a much better choice than a fully synthetic product.

Here are some recommendations and examples for good supplements and brands, especially with specialized combined ingredients, to use for beneficial health and wellness.

Multivitamin formulas and more:

The People's Chemist Daily Dose Nature's Multi-Vitamin with Turmeric 30-60 day supply for $34.95. Purchase online through the People's Chemist. There is an available website that you can go to and purchase this item as well as check out other nutritional supplements. Search for yourself at: www.thepeopleschemist.com

The People's Chemist, Shane Ellison, has written some great books and created some powerful nutritional supplements. He is a medicinal chemist with a master's in chemistry. Mr. Ellison has a great story and testimony of how and why he became a natural chemist as well as how he changed his own health and body.

His supplements are all-natural in their purest form with absolutely nothing synthetic added. Mr. Ellison's products and ingredients seem to be wisely put together and backed by studies as well as testimonies.

Here are some more examples of good quality Multivitamins:

NOW Foods ECO Green Multi with 90 vcaps for $11.77 through Swanson Vitamins

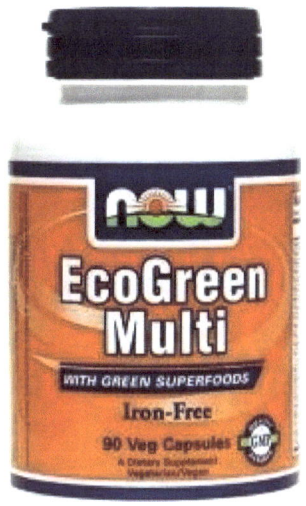

NOW Foods True Balance hi-potency multi with 120 caps for $13.99 through Nutrition Express

NOW Foods Adam Superior Men's Multi with 180 sgels for $25.83 through Swanson Vitamins

NOW Foods Eve Superior Women's Multi with 120 vcaps for $20.31 through Swanson Vitamins

Good quality examples of Whole Food Prenatal Multivitamins to choose from:

New Chapter Prenatal Multivitamin with 96 tabs for $27.95 through Nutrition Express

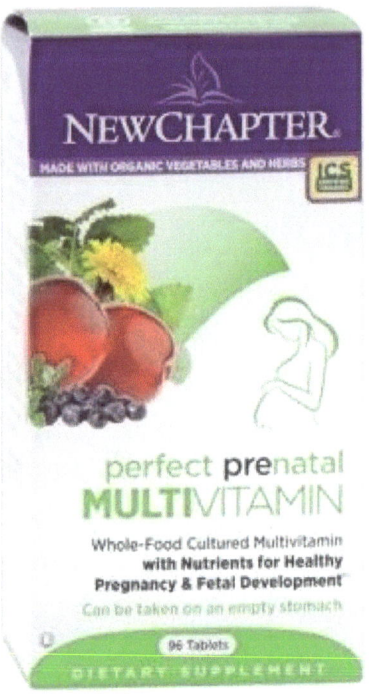

NOW Foods Prenatal Gels + DHA with 90 sgels for $14.49 through Nutrition Express

Here's a good quality example of a prostate formula for men to choose:

NOW Foods Prostate Health Clinical Strength with 90 sgels for $22.73 through Swanson Vitamins

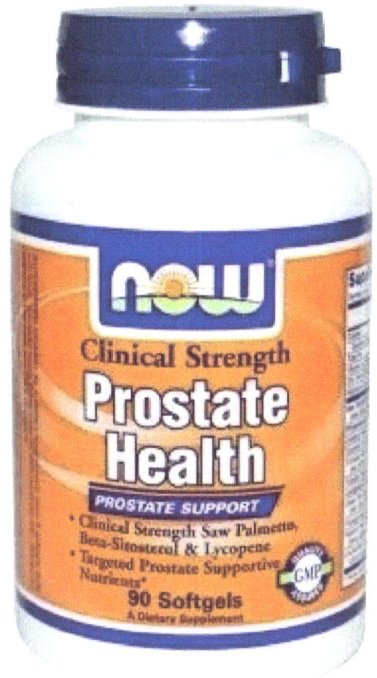

Good quality examples of Immune support and Antioxidant formulas to choose from:

Kyolic makes a great specialized supplement to support and boost your immune system for $9.49 through Nutrition Express called Kyolic Immune Formula.

It contains aged garlic, Vitamin C, Astragalus Extract, Oregano Extract and Olive Leaf Extract. It also contains a premium mushroom complex providing Shiitake, Maitake, Poria Cocos, Reishi and Agaricus.

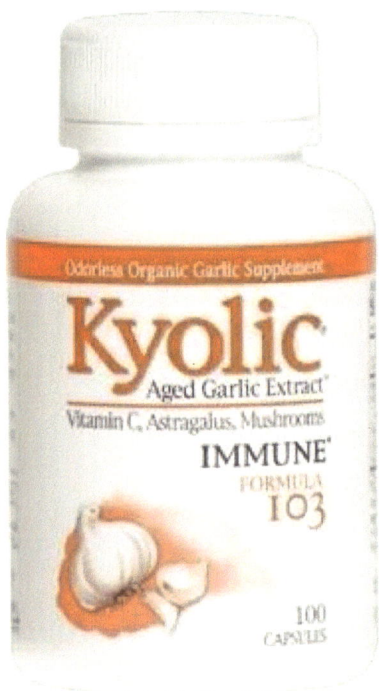

Vitamin C is always a good solid supplement to use, so here is a good one to choose:NOW Foods C-1000 (1000 mg) with 100 Mg Bioflavonoids with 250 Caps for $14.99 through Nutrition Express. You can also get this same product in 90 tabs for $10.80 also through Nutrition Express

Jarrow Formulas Antioxidant Optimizer with 90 vtabs for $16.77

Nature's Way Antioxidant Formula with 60 tabs for $14.39 through Swanson Vitamins

Jarrow Formulas CarotenAll with 60 sgels for $16.49 through Swanson Vitamins

Swanson Full Spectrum Cacao (Raw Cocoa) with 60 caps 400 mg for $2.99 through Swanson Vitamins

Swanson Organic Cocoa Polyphenols Extract with 30 organic vcaps 700 mg containing extract providing a minimum 10% total polyphenols and minimum 3% cocoa flavanols for $19.99 through Swanson Vitamins

Jarrow Formulas Blackcurrant Freeze-Dried Extract with 60 caps 200 mg for $15.37 through Swanson Vitamins

Both natural coffee and cocoa have become well known for their health benefits. Many times I'll drink decaf coffee, but I'll add a heaping teaspoon or more of 100% pure unsweetened cocoa and raw honey as a sweetener. This combination really works good for me. I have tried cocoa in caffeinated coffee several times when I need the extra caffeine and boost, but it's really too strong for me.

Good quality examples of joint, Omega Fatty Acid and healthy oil formulas to choose from:

Lindberg ArthRenew with 210 caps for $27.99 through Nutrition Express

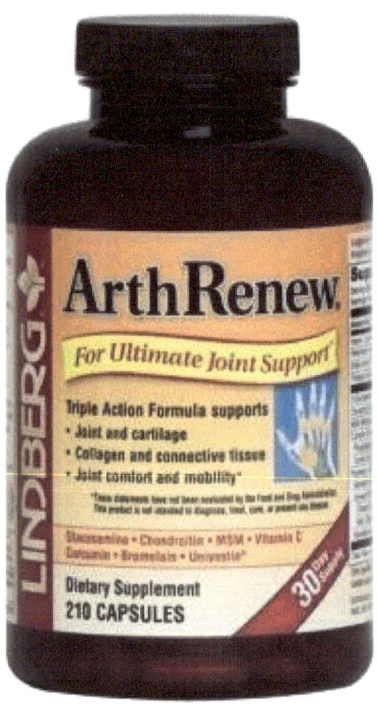

Nature's Way Hydraplenish Hyaluronic Acid with 60 vcaps for $11.59 through Swanson Vitamins

ProSource Extra Strength Joint Command with 150 caps for $23.95. Purchase online through ProSource.net

Swanson ActiJoint Plus with Krill Oil containing 60 sgels for $19.99

Jarrow Formulas PhosphOmega with 30 sgels 1000 mg of combined ingredients for $11.32 through Swanson Vitamins

Jarrow Formulas Bone-Up with 120 caps for $11.87 through Swanson Vitamins

Swanson Full Spectrum Boswellia and Curcumin with 60 caps providing 300 mg for each of these powerful ingredients. Purchase online through Swanson Vitamins for $4.49. I've used this product and it works really well at such a great price.

Good quality examples of B-Vitamin formulas to choose from:

Jarrow Formulas B-Right Optimized B-Complex with 100 vcaps for $11.79 through Swanson Vitamins

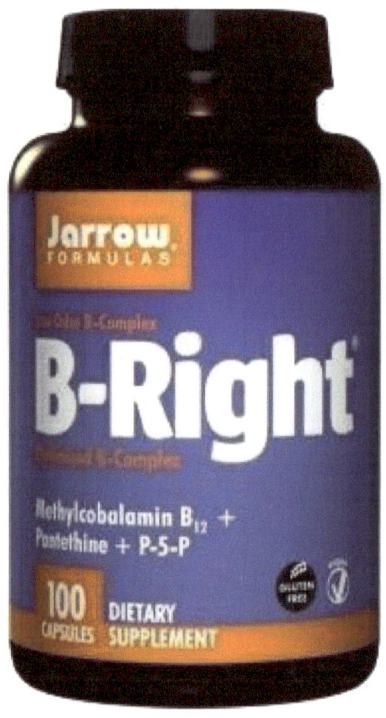

Solaray Mega B-Stress Two-Stage with 60 caps for $6.29 through Swanson Vitamins

Magnesium is another very important mineral that many people may not be getting enough of according to some recent studies. Here's a good example of a high quality magnesium supplement:

Jarrow Formulas Magnesium Optimizer Magnesium Malate with 100 tabs 100 mg plus more for $7.09 through Swanson Vitamins

Here are some final examples of beneficial supplements to research, look for and maybe try, which could give you very positive results:

Indole-3-Carbinol (Powerful antioxidant & supports healthy hormone balance)

Astragalus Extract (Promotes liver health & boost immune system)

Ubiquinol (Raises levels of CoQ10 in the bloodstream promoting energy)

CLA-Conjugated Linoleic Acid (Patented fatty acid that promotes lean muscle and decreases body fat)

L-Methionine (Promotes healthy liver and antioxidant protection)

L-Leucine (Aids in muscle recovery and increases energy as well as endurance)

L-Lysine (Boost immune system and fights stress)

L-Glutamine (Promotes brain health and boost immune system as well as muscle recovery)

Glutathione (Boost immune system and fights free radicals)

Boron (Provides support for strong health bones)

Mucuna pruriens (Promotes feel-good hormones as well as sexual and mental health)

St. John's Wort (Promotes emotional wellness and mental health)

Pure MSM (Promotes joint and cartilage health)

Royal Jelly (Food of the queen bee that boost energy, immune health and vitality)

GABA (Fights stress as well as promotes brain and physical health)

Colostrum (Boost immune system and supports muscle recovery)

L-Tyrosine (Supports vital brain chemicals and promotes mental health)

Holy Basil Extract (Fights stress and promotes relaxation)

Aloe Vera Gels (Provides beneficial nutrients and supports digestive health)

Green tea extract (Powerful free radical fighting antioxidant that also supports weight loss)

Borage oil (Rich source of GLA that supports skin and joints as well as menstrual health)

Flaxseed oil (Rich in omega fatty acids and supports cardiovascular health. Contains potential cancer fighting properties)

Acetyl L-Carnitine (Supports brain and cognitive health as well as provides antioxidant protection)

Beet Root (Supports digestive, blood and liver health)

Celery Seed Extract (Promotes wellness, digestive and joint health. Contains potential cancer fighting ability)

Fenugreek Extract (Supports healthy blood sugar, cholesterol and sex-drive levels. Promotes lactate production for breast-feeding mothers)

Maca Root (Promotes stamina, vitality and sexual health)

Black Walnut (Promotes digestive tract health, well-being and contains potential cancer fighting properties)

Horse Chestnut (Promotes healthy blood circulation, especially in the legs)

Pomegranate Extract (Powerful antioxidant that promotes liver and cardiovascular health. Contains potential cancer fighting properties)

Graviola (Promotes healthy cell growth and contains potential cancer fighting properties. Be careful with the dose when taking this and make sure you are medically able to use this supplement)

CoQ10 (Supports the production of ATP-energy)

Beta-Sitosterol (Good for men and women. Supports cardiovascular, prostate, menopause and immune health. Supports sexual health, vitality and may even slow hair loss)

On an ending note....

Four strong long-time high quality brands that I prefer are NOW Foods, Jarrow Formulas, Nature's Way and Solaray. However, Swanson brand products under Swanson Vitamins offer some really decent quality supplements with unbeatable prices. They all support and promote high standard testing as well as clinical trial studies.

There are many companies and brands out there that have created some very high quality nutritional supplements. You just got to know what your looking for and be careful before you buy, because your health may depend on it.

Nutritional supplements have their place in the world and are here to stay. Natural supplements in their purest form may even one day hold the key to the cure for cancer.

END